# Chronic obstructive pulmonary d

## Second Edition

# Chronic obstructive pulmonary disease

Second Edition

**Peter J Barnes**, MA, DM, DSc, FRCP
Professor of Thoracic Medicine
National Heart and Lung Institute
Imperial School of Medicine
London, UK

**Simon Godfrey**, MD, PhD, FRCP
Director, Institute of Pulmonology
Hadassah University Hospital
Jerusalem, Israel

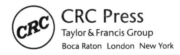

CRC Press
Taylor & Francis Group
Boca Raton London New York

CRC Press is an imprint of the
Taylor & Francis Group, an **informa** business

CRC Press
Taylor & Francis Group
6000 Broken Sound Parkway NW, Suite 300
Boca Raton, FL 33487-2742

© 2000 by Taylor & Francis Group, LLC
CRC Press is an imprint of Taylor & Francis Group, an Informa business

No claim to original U.S. Government works

**Visit the Taylor & Francis Web site at**
**http://www.taylorandfrancis.com**

**and the CRC Press Web site at**
**http://www.crcpress.com**

# Contents

# What is COPD?

## DEFINITIONS

Chronic obstructive pulmonary disease (COPD), sometimes called chronic obstructive airways disease, is a major health burden and accounts for 10% of all working days lost and over 15 000 deaths each year in the United Kingdom (UK). COPD is the third commonest cause of death in the UK and USA.

**Chronic simple bronchitis** – is defined by a productive cough on most days for at least 3 months for at least 2 consecutive years and cannot be attributed to other pulmonary or cardiac causes. It is a consequence of mucous hyperplasia and is not necessarily related to airway obstruction.

**Chronic obstructive bronchitis** – is due to obstruction of peripheral airways as a result of an inflammatory response (bronchiolitis).

**Emphysema** – is a pathological diagnosis characterized by destruction of alveolar walls, resulting in abnormal enlargement of airspaces and loss of lung elasticity, with consequent obstruction of peripheral airways.

**COPD** – is defined physiologically as chronic airflow obstruction and may be due to a mixture of emphysema and peripheral airway obstruction from chronic obstructive bronchitis. Extensive pulmonary damage occurs before the patient is aware of symptoms, such as exertional dyspnoea, owing to the slowly progressive nature of the airflow obstruction and various coping manoeuvres. There may be a small degree of reversibility in airway obstruction (<15%), in contrast to the greater than 15% reversibility and variability in the airflow obstruction in asthma.

**Chronic hypoxia** – This occurs late in COPD and may result in *pulmonary hypertension* and right heart failure (*cor pulmonale*).

**Asthma** differs from COPD in that there is a greater reversibility both spontaneously and with treatment with bronchodilators or steroids. Some patients with asthma have progressive irreversible airflow obstruction and therefore have a form of COPD, and some patients may have coexistent asthma and COPD. There is still uncertainty as to whether atopy predisposes to the development of COPD in cigarette smokers (the 'Dutch hypothesis').

## EPIDEMIOLOGY

Approximately 15–20% of middle-aged men and 10% of women in the UK report chronic cough and sputum. Most chronic smokers develop mucus hypersecretion.

COPD is diagnosed in approximately 4% of men and 2% of women over 45 years. Approximately 6% of deaths in men and 4% in women are due to COPD. There is a worldwide increase in COPD due to increased cigarette smoking in developing countries and an increasing life-span in developed countries.

COPD is an important cause of time off work, accounting for 9% of all certified sickness absences in the UK.

## CAUSES

**Cigarette smoking** – is by far the commonest cause worldwide. Active smoking causes both mucus hypersecretion and chronic airflow obstruction. Cessation of smoking reduces mucus hypersecretion and reduces the rate of decline in lung function. Passive smoking is weakly associated with COPD, mainly via an effect on lung growth during fetal development.

**Air pollution** – particularly with sulphur dioxide and particulates (black smoke), is associated with chronic simple bronchitis and COPD.

**Occupational exposure** – exposure to fumes and dusts may be important and interacts with cigarette smoking. Exposure to cadmium is associated with emphysema.

**Chest infection** – during the first year of life is associated with COPD in later life, but there is little evidence that subsequent chest infections are important.

**Diet** – may be important, because small-for-dates babies have an increased risk of development of COPD in later life. Low dietary intake of antioxidant vitamins (A, C, and E) is also associated with increased risk of COPD.

**Genetic factors** – may be important; there are several forms of antiprotease deficiency which predispose to the development of emphysema. Genetic factors may explain why only 15% of smokers develop COPD.

## PATHOLOGY

*Chronic obstructive bronchitis* is due to hyperplasia of submucosal glands and increased numbers of goblet cells in the epithelium (Fig. 1).

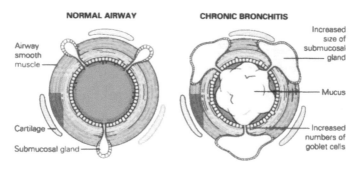

**Figure 1** *Normal and chronic bronchitic airways.*

*Chronic bronchitis* is associated with structural narrowing of small airways (bronchioles) as a result of chronic inflammatory changes. These inflammatory changes consist of activated T lymphocytes and macrophages. In larger airways there is evidence of neutrophilic inflammation, as judged by increased numbers of neutrophils in the sputum.

*Emphysema* is due to enzymatic destruction of the alveolar walls. Different patterns of emphysema are observed: centriancinar emphysema radiates from the terminal bronchiole, whereas panacinar emphysema involves more widespread destruction. Large airspaces from bullae. Emphysema results in airway obstruction caused by loss of elastic recoil; intrapulmonary airways close more readily during expiration (Fig. 2).

*COPD* is associated with both small airway obstruction and emphysema (Fig. 2), although it is likely that in most patients emphysema is the most important mechanism of chronic airflow obstruction, with the loss of peribronchial alveolar attachments.

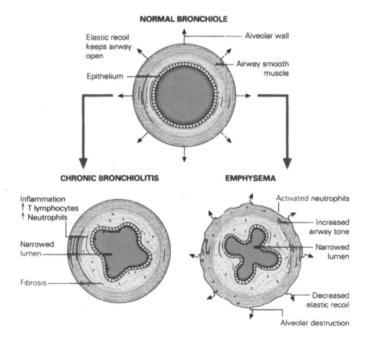

**Figure 2** *Peripheral airways in normal/chronic bronchiolitis/emphysema individuals.*

## MECHANISMS

### Mucus hypersecretion

This occurs as a result of cigarette smoking or exposure to other inhaled irritants. The mechanism probably involves activation of sensory nerve endings in the airways with reflex (local peptidergic and spinal cholinergic) increase in mucus secretion and direct stimulatory effects of enzymes such as neutrophil elastase and chymase. With time there is hyperplasia of submucosal glands and proliferation of goblet cells under the influence of unidentified growth factors.

### Small airways obstruction

This probably results from a chronic inflammatory process induced by irritants and characterized by neutrophil infiltration, as a result of the release of chemotactic factors, such as interleukin-8 and leukotriene $B_4$ from macrophages. This may then result in secretion of fibrogenic mediators, leading to fibrosis of peripheral airways.

### Protease–antiprotease imbalance

*Emphysema* is due to an imbalance between proteases (which digest elastin and other structural proteins in the alveolar wall) and antiproteases (which protect against this attack).

The major antiprotease in lungs is $\alpha_1$-*antitrypsin* (also known as $\alpha_1$-protease inhibitor) which is mainly derived from plasma. Inheritance of homozygous $\alpha_1$-antitrypsin deficiency may result in severe emphysema, particularly in cigarette smokers, but this genetic disease accounts for less than 1% of cases of COPD. $\alpha_1$-antitrypsin is not the only antiprotease; $\alpha_1$-*antichymotrypsin* and tissue inhibitors of matrix is also present in the lungs. Heterozygous individuals who have lower than normal levels of $\alpha_1$-antitrypsin have an increased risk of COPD.

*Secretory leukocyte protease inhibitor* (SLPI) may also be important. It is derived from airway epithelial cells and therefore provides a local protective mechanism.

Cigarette smoking may predispose to emphysema by stimulating alveolar macrophages to recruit neutrophils, via the release of chemotactic mediators, into the lung. The neutrophils then release proteases such as neutrophil elastase and cathespin (Fig. 3). *Neutrophil elastase* appears to be the most important protease and may result in alveolar wall damage, mucus hypersecretion and impaired mucociliary clearance. Smoking may also reduce the activity of $\alpha_1$-antitrypsin. The reason that only a proportion of smokers (approximately 15%) develop emphysema may relate to levels of antiprotease inhibitors in the lung. These may be determined by mutations in the genes for antiproteases (genetic polymorphism).

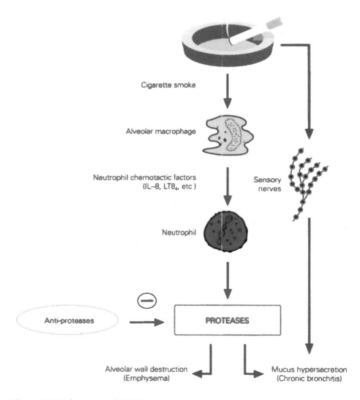

**Figure 3** *Mechanisms of COPD.*

For example, a mutation of the $\alpha_1$-antitrypsin gene has been described in approximately 10% of emphysema patients and appears to occur in the regulatory site of the gene, suggesting that control of $\alpha_1$-antitrypsin production may be defective, perhaps during an acute respiratory infection.

## COMPLICATIONS

Progressive airflow obstruction may lead to *respiratory failure* with hypoxia and hypercapnia.

Chronic hypoxia may also result in *pulmonary hypertension* due to sustained hypoxic vasoconstriction, which results in remodelling of the pulmonary circulation. This may result in progressive strain on the right heart, eventually leading to failure (*cor pulmonale*).

# Clinical features and investigation

The term COPD implies in adults the common type of chronic lung disease with airways obstruction usually related to smoking, and excludes other generalized conditions such as asthma, or localized conditions such as bronchiectasis. The patient may of course have more than one lung disease at the same time. For example, COPD and carcinoma of the lung may well coexist in a heavy smoker and some patients may have COPD and asthma.

The clinical features of COPD are usually quite straightforward and care should be taken to evaluate those features of the illness that are not typical.

## SYMPTOMS TYPICAL OF COPD

- History of heavy smoking for many years – often >25 pack years*
- Cough and sputum production for many years
- Cough often present only on waking at first; later cough occurs throughout the day
- Sputum usually mucoid – becomes purulent with exacerbation of disease, but not excessive
- Cough and sputum often worse in winter due to infection
- Insidious onset of breathlessness on exertion with wheezing or tightness of chest
- Some develop increasingly severe exacerbations of disease leading to chronic respiratory failure and heart failure – the 'blue bloater' type of COPD
- Others have little or no sputum or hypoxia at rest, but breathlessness and wheezing is severe and emphysema is prominent – the 'pink puffer' type of COPD. These patients are commonly underweight
- Most patients with COPD present with a mixed pattern rather than the 'blue bloater' or 'pink puffer' extremes

* Pack year = packs (of 20 cigarettes) smoked per day X years of smoking

## SYMPTOMS NOT TYPICAL OF COPD

- Haemoptysis – can occur due to COPD alone, but its appearance in such a patient suggests the possibility of malignancy, which must be carefully sought
- Seasonal exacerbations in spring or summer are more likely in asthma
- Excellent response to bronchodilators or steroids with definite symptom-free intervals is suggestive of asthma, not COPD
- Continuous expectoration of purulent sputum is more typical of bronchiectasis than COPD
- Breathlessness without productive cough or wheezing is more typical of cardiac disease or of other lung diseases such as interstitial pulmonary fibrosis

## PHYSICAL EXAMINATION

The typical patient with established COPD shows some or all of the following features:

- Large, barrel-shaped chest
- Prominent accessory respiratory muscles in neck
- Low, flat diaphragm causing costal margin retractions on inspiration
- Diminished breath sounds, distant heart sounds
- Prolonged expiration with generalized wheezing predominantly on expiration
- Depressed liver, which is not enlarged
- The 'blue bloater' type of COPD patient may also have:
  cyanosis at rest or mild exertion
  oedema of ankles
  crackles at lung bases
  loud second heart sound in pulmonary area (difficult to hear in COPD)
- The 'pink puffer' type of COPD patient may also have:
  expiratory pursed-lip breathing (auto-PEEP)
  thin body build
  tendency to lean forward over a support to assist breathing

*'Clubbing' is not a feature of COPD and suggests either malignancy, bronchiectasis, or some other type of lung disease.*

## INVESTIGATIONS

Any patient presenting with a history of cough, sputum production and breathlessness requires certain basic investigations which may in turn suggest the need for further investigations.

## Chest X-ray

In mild COPD the plain chest radiograph may well be normal, but with advancing disease – and in particular with the appearance of significant amounts of emphysema – changes occur, and include:

- Large volume lungs
- Low, flat diaphragm
- Thin heart shadow
- Enlarged retrosternal air space

When *emphysema* is prominent there is loss of fine vascular markings, and bullae may appear, especially at the apices.

When *cor pulmonale* occurs the hilar vasculature may become prominent, and the heart may enlarge – especially in the anteroposterior direction.

With *infections* there may be localized infiltrates in the lungs. These should disappear with treatment.

The following features on a plain chest radiograph are *not* consistent with a diagnosis of uncomplicated COPD and should raise the possibility of an alternative diagnosis:

- Persistent localized infiltrate
- Persistent atelectasis
- Hilar node enlargement
- Parenchymal nodules or masses
- Pleural disease
- Interstitial infiltrates

## CT scan of lungs

Although it is perfectly possible to diagnose and manage COPD without performing a CT scan of the lungs, there are a number of good reasons why this may be indicated one or more times as the disease progresses:

- Most patients with COPD are heavy smokers and a small carcinoma may be difficult to diagnose on a plain chest radiograph

- It may be impossible to distinguish between simple infectious exacerbations of COPD and the appearance of malignancy on a plain radiograph
- The extent of emphysema is best judged by a high-resolution scan CT (Fig. 4)
- Complications of COPD such as pulmonary thromboembolism and pulmonary artery thrombosis can be detected by a CT scan with contrast injection – especially by the spiral (continuous) CT technique

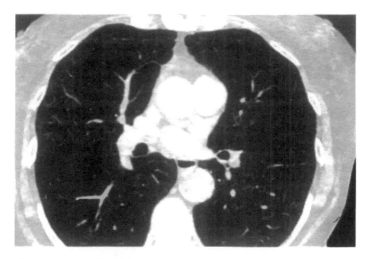

**Figure 4** *CT scan of emphysema.*

## Lung function

The hallmark of COPD is chronic airflow obstruction, which is largely irreversible. The obstruction is particularly marked in the smaller airways, owing to the pathological changes of chronic obstructive bronchitis and the loss of support of their walls due to emphysema. These small airways close off during expiration, trapping gas and increasing resting lung volume (functional residual capacity, FRC) and residual volume (RV). Emphysema may also result in an increase in total lung capacity (TLC) and loss of the alveolar surface area available for gas exchange. There are various tests that are useful in evaluating lung function in COPD:

## Spirometry

The simplest and most useful measure of airways obstruction is obtained by having the patient perform a forced expiration from TLC and recording the spirogram as either a flow–volume or a volume–time plot (Fig. 5).

In COPD the following changes are to be expected:

- *Forced expired volume in 1 second* (FEV$_1$) – always reduced, with progressively greater reduction as disease advances. FEV$_1$ is the most useful test to assess the severity and progression of COPD (Table 1).

| Severity | FEV$_1$ (% predicted) |
|----------|-----------------------|
| Mild | ⩾70 |
| Moderate | 50–69 |
| Severe | <50 |

**Table 1** *Airways obstruction and forced expired volume in 1 second.*

- *Forced vital capacity* (FVC) – initially normal, but reduced as disease progresses.

- *FEV$_1$/FVC ratio* – classically used by respiratory physicians to evaluate COPD – always less than the normal adult value of about 80%, and becoming worse as disease progresses; may not accurately reflect very severe COPD, since FVC is then also reduced.

- *Peak expiratory flow* (PEF) – a crude estimate of lung function, reflecting larger airway function and very effort-dependent – reduced roughly in proportion to disease severity. Not as useful in COPD as in asthma, as it may be relatively well preserved in emphysema.

- *Maximum mid-expiratory flow* (MMEF) – reflects primarily small airways function and is markedly reduced in patients with COPD.

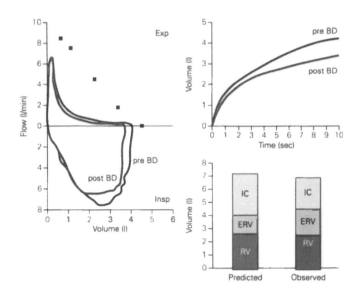

| | Predicted | Baseline | Post BD |
|---|---|---|---|
| FEV₁ (litres) | 3.34 | 1.53 | 1.43 |
| FVC (litres) | 4.24 | 4.17 | 3.43 |
| FEV₁/FVC (%) | 76 | 37 | 42 |
| PEF (litres/min) | 8.38 | 6.69 | 6.73 |
| MMEF (litres/min) | 4.46 | 0.45 | 0.34 |
| TLC (litres) | 6.98 | 6.59 | |
| FRC (litres) | 3.22 | 4.52 | |
| RV (litres) | 2.40 | 2.43 | |
| SVC = ERV + IC (litres) | 4.23 | 4.16 | |
| SG$_{aw}$ (cmH$_2$O$^{-1}$. sec$^{-1}$) | 0.20 | 0.10 | |
| DLCO (ml/min per mmHg) | 28.6 | 31.6 | |
| DL/Va | 4.09 | 4.72 | |

**Figure 5** *Lung function in a 60-year-old man with COPD showing a very obstructive pattern on the flow–volume and volume–time plots with no improvement on inhaling a bronchodilator (BD). The lung volumes show mild hyperinflation. Diffusing capacity was normal.*

The effect of inhaling a bronchodilator on spirometry is usually minimal, with a less than 20% increase in $FEV_1$, but some patients may have a better response, even if they never reach normal values (Fig. 6).

### Lung volumes and airway resistance

Spirometry alone is often adequate to evaluate the abnormality of lung mechanics in COPD. However, when the disease is severe, when there is doubt about the diagnosis, or when it is important to know the extent of the emphysema (e.g. when considering volume reduction surgery or lung transplantation) further investigation is required.

The whole-body plethysmograph is a closed chamber in which the patient sits while respiratory flow and pressure are recorded at the mouth along with pressure changes in the chamber. By application of Boyle's Law it is possible to measure absolute lung volumes and the resistance of the whole airway from alveoli to mouth (Figs 5 and 6):

- *Total lung capacity* (TLC) – normal to modest increase in most COPD; may be markedly increased in patients with predominant emphysema.

- *Residual volume* (RV) – invariably increased, owing to gas trapping; RV/TLC ratio always >40%.

- *Resting lung volume* (FRC) – increased as with RV, but a less reliable measurement.

- *Expiratory reserve volume* (ERV) – the difference between FRC and RV – mild to moderate reduction n COPD.

- *Inspiratory capacity* (IC) – the difference between TLC and FRC – usually reduced in COPD.

- *Slow vital capacity* (SVC) – the size of the largest breath (not forced) that can be taken – the sum of ERV and IC – reduced in more severe COPD.

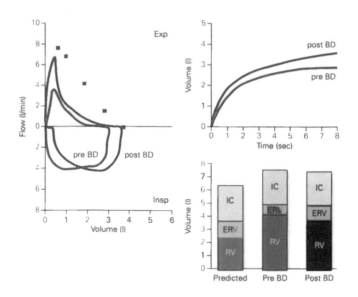

| | Predicted | Baseline | Post BD |
|---|---|---|---|
| FEV$_1$ (litres) | 2.95 | 1.62 | 1.97 |
| FVC (litres) | 3.72 | 2.95 | 3.55 |
| FEV$_1$/FVC (%) | 79 | 55 | 55 |
| PEF (litres/min) | 7.82 | 46 | 89 |
| MMEF (litres/min) | 4.12 | 0.87 | 1.52 |
| TLC (litres) | 6.26 | 7.45 | 7.37 |
| FRC (litres) | 3.36 | 4.86 | 4.76 |
| RV (litres) | 2.28 | 4.20 | 3.68 |
| SVC = ERV + IC (litres) | 3.99 | 3.25 | 3.69 |
| SG$_{aw}$ (cmH$_2$O $^1$. sec $^1$) | 0.20 | 0.04 | 0.09 |
| DLCO (ml/min per mmHg) | 26.1 | 15.0 | |
| DL/Va | 4.11 | 3.18 | |

**Figure 6** *Lung function in another 60-year-old man with COPD showing a moderate response to inhaled bronchodilator with improvement in airway obstruction and lung volumes. The patient had quite severe hyperinflation and reduced diffusing capacity, suggesting that emphysema was an important element in his COPD.*

- *Airways resistance* ($R_{aw}$) – reflects chiefly larger and medium-sized airways and usually increased in COPD. Commonly expressed as its reciprocal and related to the thoracic gas volume ($V_{tg}$) at which resistance was measured.

$1/R_{aw} = G_{aw}$ (airway conductance) – usually reduced
$SG_{aw} = G_{aw}/V_{tg}$ (specific airway conductance) – usually reduced

Lung volumes can also be measured by inert gas dilution methods, but this is unreliable in all but the mildest COPD since the uneven ventilation prevents good mixing of the marker gas with the gas in the lungs.

### Arterial blood gases

COPD is invariably accompanied by some degree of ventilation/perfusion (V/Q), mismatching of which results in arterial hypoxia when room air is breathed. In some patients there is also a degree of respiratory failure resulting in an increase in arterial $Pa,CO_2$. In COPD patients with chronic respiratory failure there should be metabolic compensation with an elevated base excess (or bicarbonate) and relatively normal pH. Pulse oximetry measures oxygen saturation ($Sa,O_2$), but is not a good guide for diagnostic purposes, since it only indicates oxygenation and does not indicate the changes in $Pa,CO_2$; it may be useful for following the development of hypoxia as the disease advances. If $Sa,O_2$ is less than 92% blood gas tensions should be measured (Table 2).

| | $Pa,O_2$ mmHg (kPa) | $Pa,CO_2$ mmHg (kPa) | Base excess (mmol) | pH |
|---|---|---|---|---|
| 'Typical' COPD not in respiratory failure | 70 (9.3) | 40 (5 3) | 0 | 7.40 |
| 'Typical' COPD in acute respiratory failure | 45 (6.0) | 60 (8 0) | −3 | 7.25 |
| 'Typical' COPD in chronic respiratory failure | 50 (6.7) | 55 (7 3) | +8 | 7.40 |

Table 2 *Arterial blood gas tensions.*

## Gas transfer (diffusing capacity)

In most patients with COPD gas transfer is relatively well preserved, but when emphysema is marked the surface area for gas exchange is reduced and, typically, there is a fall in the transfer factor ('diffusing capacity': DLCO) of carbon monoxide (and similarly of oxygen) both in absolute terms and especially in relation to the increased alveolar volume (transfer coefficient: $K$CO or DLCO/Va).

## Exercise testing

Some patients with mild COPD may have little or no disturbance of blood gases at rest, and hypoxia only appears on exercise. In others with more marked disease, the decision as to whether to recommend supplemental oxygen should be made with the help of an objective evaluation of the degree of effort limitation. There are several exercise protocols in use:

**Six minute walk** – In this test the patient is encouraged to walk as far as possible at their own pace for 6 minutes and the total distance walked is noted. In a more advanced version of this test the patient is fitted with a pulse oximeter and oxygen saturation is measured throughout the test. The distance covered correlates well with lung function (diffusing capacity) but not with oxygen saturation during the walk. In a typical COPD patient with an $FEV_1$ of about 1 litre or 40% predicted, the 6 minute walk distance would be about 400 metres. There is considerable intersubject variability, which depends to some degree on emotional state, expectations and motivation. It is a valuable and simple index for following progression of the disease in the individual patient

**Shuttle test** – This involves walking round two markers and is easier to conduct in a hospital setting than the 6 minute walk test

**Progressive ergometer stress test** – In this test the patient exercises on a cycle ergometer (or treadmill) with a progressively increasing workload until they are unable to continue further. A number of parameters can be measured which reflect the nature and severity of the disturbed physiology. These include:

- Maximum oxygen uptake – reduced in relation to severity of COPD
- Minute ventilation – increased in relation to severity of COPD
- Breathing reserve (maximum voluntary ventilation – maximum exercise ventilation) – reduced it the patient is limited by ventilation
- Estimated dead space – increased due to ventilation/perfusion mismatching

- Oxygen saturation – falls with increasing workload
- Heart rate – normal unless there is cardiac involvement
- Oxygen pulse (oxygen uptake/heart rate) – reduced if there is cardiac involvement

Note: before an exercise test of any kind is undertaken, it should be ensured that:

- The patient is in a stable state
- There is no coincident ischaemic heart disease
- There is no recent thromboembolism
- There is no cor pulmonale

Oxygenation should always be documented by pulse oximetry or arterial blood gases during an exercise test.

## Sleep studies

Many patients with significant COPD underventilate during sleep and worsen the existing ventilation/perfusion imbalance or respiratory failure. This causes further hypoxia and may initiate or aggravate pulmonary hypertension and right heart failure (cor pulmonale). A formal sleep study with polysomnography may be indicated in those suspected of having central of obstructive sleep apnoea, but for many patients it is sufficient to perform overnight monitoring of oxygenation with pulse oximetry. The greater the proportion of sleeping time spent with a saturation of less than 90%, the greater the risk of cor pulmonale. Patients without significant hypoxia when awake are unlikely to suffer as a result of desaturation during sleep, but should this cause problems then supplemental oxygen therapy during sleep may be needed.

## Haematology/biochemistry

Blood tests, other than arterial blood gas measurements, are of limited importance in the investigation and management of COPD, but may be indicated from time to time.

- *Polycythaemia* is an indication of chronic hypoxia and is most common in the 'blue bloater' type of COPD.

- Electrolyte imbalance may occur in patients with cor pulmonale, especially in those treated with diuretics in whom *hypokalaemia* may be a problem.

- Estimation of $\alpha_1$-antitrypsin levels is indicated in the initial evaluation of a patient with COPD, especially if the patient is young and emphysema is prominent.

- Estimation of $\alpha_1$-antitrypsin phenotype by genetic Pi typing is indicated if the $\alpha_1$-antitrypsin levels are very low or if a variant of the disorder is suspected.

## Trial of steroids

COPD by definition is a form of obstructive lung disease with a relatively poor degree of reversibility; in these patients the functional response to an inhaled bronchodilator is rarely dramatic. However, there are also some patients with chronic asthma whose response to bronchodilator inhalation is poor, and it is important to distinguish the conditions as the management is quite different. For this reason it is probably worth performing a trial of corticosteroid therapy in all patients with significant obstructive lung disease unless a definite diagnosis has already been established. In order to perform this trial:

- Estimate airways obstruction (spirometry) before and after bronchodilator use
- Measure lung volume (plethysmography)
- Measure arterial blood gases
- Monitor a 6 minute walk or similar exercise test
- Give prednisolone 30 or 40 mg daily for 2 weeks
- Repeat all lung function and exercise measurements

A dramatic improvement in all parameters to within the normal range suggests that the diagnosis is asthma, not COPD.

A modest improvement but not to normal may be an indication that corticosteroid therapy could help the patient with COPD. No improvement suggests that corticosteroids have no place in the management and may simply produce unwanted side-effects. Beware the euphoric effect of corticosteroids, which may make the patient feel better in the absence of any objective improvement.

## Bronchial provocation tests

The hallmark of bronchial asthma is bronchial hyperreactivity in which the airways of the asthmatic constrict when stimulated with various chemical or physical agents at a much lower level than those which stimulate normal subjects. Patients with COPD display bronchial hyperreactivity but this is due to geometric factors because of pre-existing airway narrowing. There are differences in the response to various agents between asthmatics and COPD patients; whereas both may respond to methacholine or histamine (direct bronchoconstrictors), only asthmatics respond to exercise or to adenosine 5'-monophosphate inhalation (indirect bronchoconstrictors). Although this is of considerable theoretical interest, bronchial provocation challenges are rarely indicated in patients with COPD.

## SPECIAL TYPES OF COPD

In some patients COPD is unrelated or only partly related to cigarette smoking, and COPD can also occur in children and young people, owing to a variety of causes.

## Deficiency of $\alpha_1$-antitrypsin

This is due to a severe reduction in antiprotease in the lung as a result of a genetic defect. This renders the lung tissue susceptible to the destructive effects of various endogenous proteases and results in severe emphysema, especially in smokers. This type of COPD appears at a much younger age (in the third or fourth decade) and may even appear in childhood. The condition is rare and only occurs in homozygous carriers of the defective genes. Heterozygotes are usually healthy.

## Cystic fibrosis

In this condition, there is a form of COPD due to a genetic defect affecting ion transport across cell membranes. This results in abnormal mucus in the airway with repeated infection and lung damage and (usually) pancreatic insufficiency with failure to thrive. Many children now live to adulthood with effective treatment, and in some genetic variants the disease may be so mild as to appear only in adult life.

## Primary ciliary dyskinesia

This disorder is due to a defect in the ultrastructure of cilia throughout the body, commonly resulting in chronic sinusitis, chronic otitis, and COPD. Males are sterile because of immotile spermatozoa. In its most extreme form there may be dextrocardia and bronchiectasis (Kartagener's syndrome), but most patients have a relatively mild type of COPD.

## Postviral bronchiolitis obliterans

This usually follows adenoviral pneumonia in childhood which produces severe damage to the small airways and varying degrees of COPD. Sometimes the disease is relatively mild, but it can persist as a severe form throughout life. Occasionally one lung is much more affected than the other and the result is a unilateral small, hyperlucent lung (McLeod's syndrome or Swyer–James syndrome). Bronchiolitis obliterans can also be acquired in adult life and is a recognized complication after transplantation of bone marrow, heart, or lung.

### DIFFERENTIAL DIAGNOSIS

The differential diagnosis of COPD compared with other types of chronic obstructive lung disease is based on the various clinical and functional parameters discussed in this section. Differentiation from the genetic disorders considered above is usually straightforward and the real problem lies in the differentiation between COPD, asthma, heart failure, and bronchiectasis in the older patient. In all these conditions cough and breathlessness are common, whereas sputum production is prominent in COPD and bronchiectasis. Sputum is characteristically purulent in bronchiectasis, but only during infective exacerbations of COPD. Haemoptysis is not uncommon in bronchiectasis and may occur in uncomplicated COPD, but should always raise the suspicion of malignancy. Differentiation from asthma is usually made with the help of tests of lung function and the differentiation from heart failure, commonly due to

| | COPD | Asthma | Heart failure | Bronchiectasis |
|---|---|---|---|---|
| Heavy smoking | usual | usually stopped smoking | not a feature | not a feature |
| Cough | early morning | night or morning | any time | any time |
| Sputum | occasionally purulent | not purulent | not a feature | usually purulent |
| Haemoptysis | occasional feature | not a feature | very occasionally | common |
| Breathlessness | all the time | only in attacks | especially lying down | not a feature |
| Malaise, confusion | with respiratory failure | with severe status asthmaticus | not uncommon in elderly | very unusual |
| Crepitations | common | uncommon | common at bases | commonly localized |
| Localized signs | uncommon | uncommon | uncommon | common |
| Generalized wheezing | common | common | uncommon | not a feature |
| Peripheral oedema | occasional | not a feature | common | not a feature |
| Obstructive spirometry | always | always in attack | unusual | unusual |
| Response to bronchodilator | poor | good | poor | poor |
| Response to corticosteroids | poor | usually good | possible harmful | unusual |

Table 3 *Differential diagnosis of COPD.*

ischaemic heart disease, is made on clinical grounds, aided by tests of cardiac function. Two or more of these conditions can occur simultaneously, but the features in Table 3 may help to make the distinction.

## NATURAL HISTORY OF COPD

Since COPD typically results from irreversible damage to the alveoli and smaller airways due to smoking there is no chance of completely curing the disease, which usually follows a slow but progressive downhill course over many years. If the patient stops smoking, the rate of decline of lung function is substantially slowed.

The typical course of COPD is characterized by:

- Breathlessness initially on exercise but later at rest
- Cough and sputum initially in morning but later all day
- Acute respiratory infections with increasing frequency, especially in winter
- Hypoxia initially on exercise but later during sleep and even at rest by day
- Chronic respiratory failure and cor pulmonale
- Terminal acute respiratory failure

Stopping smoking, appropriate medication, rehabilitation, and oxygen therapy may substantially modify the rate of progress of COPD. Patients with COPD whose lung function is relatively good ($FEV_1$ >50% predicted) when initially diagnosed and who stop smoking have a prognosis for survival similar to that of smokers who do not have COPD. During the initial evaluation and follow-up of COPD, some or all of the investigations discussed will be required from time to time. Table 4 provides a guide to those investigations which should be undertaken according to features which occur commonly in the follow-up of patients with COPD.

| Indication | Test |
|---|---|
| Routine | FEV$_1$, VC/FVC<br>Bronchodilator response<br>Chest radiograph<br>DLCO/KCO |
| Moderate/severe COPD | Lung volumes<br>Sa,O$_2$ and/or blood gases<br>ECG<br>Haemoglobin |
| Persistent purulent sputum | Sputum culture/sensitivity |
| Emphysema in young patient | $\alpha_1$-antitrypsin |
| Assessment of bullae | CT scan |
| Disproportionate breathlessness | Exercise test |
| Suspected asthma | Trial of steroids<br>PEF monitoring<br>Airway responsiveness |
| Suspected sleep apnoea | Nocturnal sleep study |

Table 4 *Indications for investigations in COPD.*

# Principles of treatment and management guidelines

Recently internationally agreed management guidelines for COPD have been published. These propose a logical approach to management, based on the best available evidence, although there is still relatively little evidence from controlled trials to dictate the optimal therapy (Fig. 7).

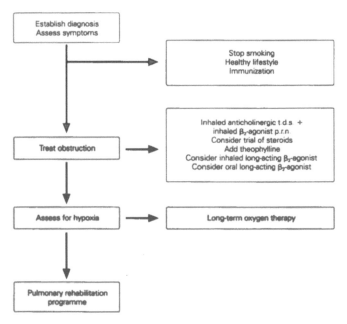

**Figure 7** *Management of COPD: summary diagram.*

Managing COPD depends upon evaluating the severity of the disorder, providing appropriate treatment and evaluating the response – usually on a long-term basis over many years.

Management should be designed:

- To reduce progression of disease
- To provide symptomatic relief and improve the quality of life
- To treat serious complications
- To avoid side-effects of therapy in achieving these aims

Management usually involves:

- Absolute cessation of smoking
- Bronchodilator treatment
- Other treatments
- Pulmonary rehabilitation

## STOPPING SMOKING

Stopping smoking is the single most beneficial management strategy and the only intervention that reduces the accelerated decline in lung function (Fig. 8). Nicotine is addictive and stopping smoking should be viewed as the treatment of drug addiction. Abrupt quitting is more successful than gradual reduction, but even after an intensive smoking cessation programme, 75% of smokers are still smoking 1 year later. There are several ways to encourage smoking cessation:

- Psychological counselling and smoking reduction clinics may be useful (addresses available from Quitline: 0171-487-3000)
- Group therapy may help some patients
- Nicotine gum doubles long-term abstinence rates
- Bupropion, a noradrenergic antidepressant is the most effective way to reduce smoking but is not available in all countries (including the UK)
- Nicotine skin patches are somewhat more successful than nicotine gum
- Nasal nicotine spray has a similar success rate to skin patches
- Hypnosis and acupuncture may be helpful in some patients

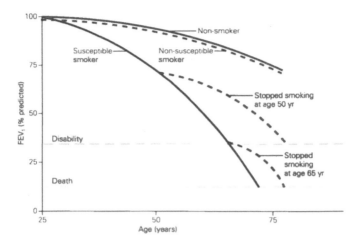

**Figure 8** *Annual decline in airway function showing accelerated decline in susceptible smokers and effects of smoking cessation.*

## BRONCHODILATORY TREATMENT

The use of bronchodilators to reduce symptoms and increase exercise tolerance is the cornerstone of management of COPD. There is no evidence that chronic bronchodilator treatment alters the natural history of COPD. In patients with COPD symptomatic improvement may not be reflected by an increase in $FEV_1$ or PEF and may be due to other actions of bronchodilators, such as:

- Reduction in pulmonary hyperinflation – making breathing more comfortable and reducing the work of breathing
- Increase in exercise tolerance
- Changes in mucociliary clearance
- Improvement in respiratory muscle function – although this is unlikely at the doses of drugs used clinically

The choice of bronchodilator may depend on individual patients. Anticholinergics appear to be more effective bronchodilators than $\beta_2$-agonists and should be given on a regular basis (e.g. ipratropium bromide 1–2 puffs (40–80 µg) three to four times daily or oxitropium bromide 200 µg t.d.s.). Short-acting $\beta_2$-agonists (e.g. salbutamol 200 µg or terbutaline 500 µg) should be used as additional treatments as required for symptom control. Inhaled long-acting $\beta_2$-agonists (salmeterol 50 µg b.d. of formoterol 12 µg b.i.d.) are useful as additional bronchodilators. Slow-release theophylline is also useful and may have particular value in reducing hyperinflation by acting on peripheral airways.

*Combination* bronchodilator inhalers with an anticholinergic and a short-acting $\beta_2$-agonist, such as Duovent (ipratropium bromide + fenoterol) and Combivent (ipratropium bromide + salbutamol) are a convenient way of giving bronchodilators.

Anticholinergics and $\beta_2$-agonists are best given by metered dose inhaler (MDI) and a large volume spacer can be helpful in increasing lung delivery in patients with more severe airway obstruction. Dry powder inhalers for anticholinergics and $\beta_2$-agonists are also available and may be preferred by some patients. Nebulizers should be reserved for patients with the most severe airflow obstruction when other forms of inhaler have failed. Drug delivery systems are described in the next chapter.

## OTHER TREATMENTS

### Prevention of infections
Lower respiratory tract infections are undoubtedly important in the initiation of COPD and in its progression. Combating these infections is therefore of great importance to management:

- *Antibiotics* should be started at the first sign of an exacerbation (see page 51) but there is no evidence that prophylactic antibiotics reduce the incidence or severity of infective exacerbations of COPD
- Prophylactic *influenza vaccination* is recommended every autumn
- *Pneumococcal vaccination* may also be indicated, but there is little evidence to date that this is useful in the long-term management of COPD

### Oxygen therapy
All patients with severe COPD are hypoxic on exercise and often at

rest or when sleeping. This hypoxia contributes to the development of pulmonary hypertension and cor pulmonale and in such patients an attempt should be made to avoid hypoxia as much as possible by providing an appropriate source of supplemental oxygen (see page 57).

## Corticosteroid therapy

While there is some evidence for airway inflammation in COPD there is no evidence that inhaled steroids prevent the progressive decline in lung function in COPD although they may reduce the severity of exacerbations. A trial of inhaled steroids is indicated in patients with severe COPD who have frequent exacerbations. Oral steroids increase the recovery from acute severe exacerbations.

## Muco regulatory therapy

Despite the attractive idea that thinning the sputum should benefit patients with COPD, the various muco regulatory agents available have not proved to be very effective so far. There is some evidence that N-acetyl cysteine is beneficial in acute exacerbations and in long-term therapy but this is likely to be due to its antioxidant effect rather than its mucolytic effect.

### PULMONARY REHABILITATION

Several non-pharmacological approaches have also been used in the management of COPD as part of a comprehensive rehabilitation programme:

- *Exercise training* to improve cardio-respiratory function may be helpful; the type of exercise does not appear to be important, and aerobic exercise or upper limb exercises are equally effective
- *Respiratory muscle training* using resistive inspiratory loading has been shown to reduce breathlessness
- *Controlled breathing techniques*, such as pursed-lip breathing and diaphragmatic breathing, result in reduced dyspnoea particularly in patients with hyperventilation
- *Nutrition* is important in patients with COPD as many patients are malnourished and underweight. Obese patients should lose weight, particularly if there are sleep disturbances. Antioxidant vitamin supplements are also indicated

- *Physiotherapy*: coughing and forced respiratory manoeuvres are helpful in expectorating sputum and reducing the likelihood of pooling and infection

## MANAGEMENT OF ASSOCIATED PROBLEMS AND END-STAGE LUNG DISEASE

With advancing COPD, serious cardiac or respiratory complications are likely to occur and require treatment:

- Treatment of heart failure due to pulmonary hypertension and cor pulmonale by the judicious use of medication and long-term oxygen therapy
- Treatment of acute or chronic respiratory failure – possibly by mechanical ventilation in hospital or at home
- Early detection and treatment of pulmonary malignancy, which is common in patients who have been very heavy cigarette smokers

In order for appropriate and timely therapy to be instituted, patients with COPD need to be reviewed periodically in a specialist pulmonary clinic, where appropriate clinical and social evaluation can be made and tests of lung function can be undertaken. The frequency of attendance depends on the severity of the condition, but ready access to the clinic should be provided between scheduled appointments.

## Clinical/social evaluation

- Quality of life, ability to work or engage in normal social activities
- Frequency of cough/sputum production
- Quantity and quality of sputum
- Degree of exercise limitation
- Breathlessness at rest
- Sleep disturbance
- Frequency of acute exacerbations of COPD
- Appearance of signs of heart failure – cor pulmonale

## Radiological evaluation

- Plain chest radiograph when any significant clinical change occurs
- CT scan of chest if there is any suspicion of malignancy
- Special radiological techniques if needed (spiral CT, angiography etc.)

## Physiological evaluation

- Spirometry ± bronchodilator at every clinic visit and at least twice/year
- Pulse oximetry at every clinic visit and whenever deterioration suspected
- Arterial blood gas measurement if respiratory failure suspected
- Full lung function tests including measurement of lung volumes, blood gases and carbon monoxide transfer factor if major clinical change occurs or if palliative surgery is contemplated
- Sleep study if there is suspicion of significant hypoxia during sleep or other sleep disturbances

## Effort tolerance

- Simple stress test – 6 minute walk, shuttle test or step test for evaluation – at least once per year

## Cardiac evaluation

- Indicated periodically to detect early signs of right heart failure (cor pulmonale) so that attempts can be made to step up treatment and improve oxygenation
- ECG performed periodically to detect signs of right ventricular enlargement or coincident ischaemic heart disease
- Echocardiography indicated to provide better information on right ventricular function and pulmonary artery pressure

# Other investigations as needed

- Sputum examination – not usually very helpful, but may give important information in patients failing to respond to usual antibiotics for acute exacerbation

- Biochemical/haematological investigations as indicated by clinical condition, e.g. diuretic therapy, suspicion of polycythaemia and chronic hypoxia
- Bronchoscopy, biopsy, etc should be used as in any other patient when there is suspicion of malignancy

## MANAGEMENT WHEN SEVERE DETERIORATION OCCURS AND OF END-STAGE LUNG DISEASE

If the clinical or functional evaluation suggests a significant deterioration or the appearance of a complication, an attempt should be made to change management in order to improve the situation or deal with the complication. This may involve:

- Trial of additional medication, change of antibiotics, trial of corticosteroids
- Home ventilation, supplemental oxygen therapy
- Start of a rehabilitation program
- In patients with severe COPD with marked emphysema who are relatively young and have no other contraindications, palliative surgery (volume reduction) may be indicated
- A single lung transplantation may be indicated in young patents with end-stage emphysema

It is important to keep these options in mind and not miss the opportunity for surgery in suitable patients by delaying the decision too long.

# Drug delivery systems

Apart from antibiotics, theophylline preparations, systemic corticosteroids, and diuretics, which are all given orally, most patients with COPD will benefit from drugs that are delivered by inhalation. These include:

- Sympathomimetic bronchodilators
- Anticholinergic bronchodilators
- Inhaled corticosteroids
- Inhaled mucolytic agents

Without any doubt many patients with COPD fail to benefit from such treatment because of an inappropriate or inefficient use of the devices available for the administration of these drugs.

There are five basic systems currently available for delivering drugs by inhalation, four of which are illustrated in Fig. 9:

- Pressurized aerosol (MDIs)
- Large volume holding chambers (spacers) for use with MDIs
- Multiple dose dry powder inhalers (DPIs)
- Wet impactor-type jet nebulizers
- Ultrasonic nebulizers

Each of these devices has advantages and disadvantages and it is important to prescribe the device most suitable for the individual patient.

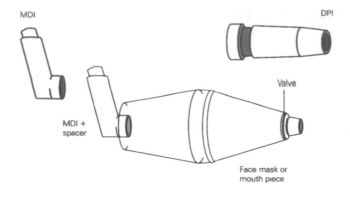

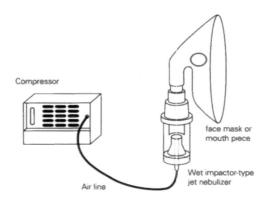

**Figure 9** *Inhalation devices.*

## METERED DOSE INHALER

The MDI contains medication mixed with a chlorofluorocarbon (CFC) propellant (to be replaced in the future by hydrofluorocarbon, which has less effect on the ozone layer) and a controlled dose is emitted as a spray when the device is activated. MDIs are available for all common bronchodilator medications.

### Advantages
- Small and portable
- Cheap
- Quick to use

### Disadvantages
- Perfect technique absolutely essential
- Unsuitable for the elderly, confused, arthritic, etc.
- Cold jet may irritate throat

### Correct technique
- Shake the inhaler
- Hold upright
- Breathe out
- Close lips around mouthpiece
- Fire device at start of slow inspiration
- Inspire to total lung capacity
- Hold breath for 10 seconds
- Breathe out

## METERED DOSE INHALER WITH SPACER

Because many patients are unable to co-ordinate well enough to use an MDI correctly, various holding chambers (spacers) have been developed which are placed between the MDI and the patient. The drug is inhaled from the chamber and co-ordination with the firing of the MDI is no longer important. Most spacers have some type of non-rebreathing valve. The type of spacer used is probably of little importance in most cases.

### Advantages

- Co-ordination unimportant
- Can be used by almost all patients
- May reduce systemic absorption of corticosteroids
- Relatively inexpensive

### Disadvantages

- Bulky and inconvenient
- Valves sometimes stick or become incompetent

### Correct technique

- Shake the inhaler
- Fix MDI upright in spacer
- Keep lips on mouthpiece
- Breathe in and out through spacer
- Fire device while taking 1–2 deep breaths
- Be sure valve is operating
- Keep spacer clean and dry

When the treatment calls for two or more doses of medication, it is important that each dose be taken separately; it is not recommended that the MDI be activated more than once per inspiration or that the spacer be loaded with several doses.

## DRY POWDER INHALER

A number of multidose devices have been developed from which the patient inhales a dry powder formulation of the drug. These do not contain CFCs and, since they are only activated by the inspiratory effort of the patient, co-ordination is not a problem, although the inhalation technique is still very important. The multidose types of powder inhalers are suitable for most patients, including those who would require a spacer in order to use an MDI. DPIs are available for sympathomimetic bronchodilators, ipratropium bromide and glucocorticoids.

### Advantages

- Co-ordination unimportant
- Can be used by almost all patients
- Small and portable
- No CFCs

### Disadvantages

- Relatively expensive
- Require rapid inspiration
- Preparing device requires a little skill

### Correct technique

- Follow instruction for preparation of device
- Breathe out
- Place lips firmly around mouthpiece
- Breathe in rapidly and deeply

One device, the Turbuhaler, appears to deliver about twice as much medication as the equivalent MDI, and the dose may need to be reduced accordingly.

## WET IMPACTOR-TYPE JET NEBULIZER

Wet impactor-type jet nebulizers produce a cloud of medication by passing a jet of compressed air over a solution of the drug. Preparations of all types of bronchodilator and one glucocorticoid (budesonide) are available for nebulization. This is the only suitable route for the inhalation of a muco regulatory agent.

### Advantages

- Co-ordination unimportant
- Can be used for all ages

### Disadvantages

- Cumbersome, noisy equipment (compressor)
- Expensive
- Treatment takes a long time (5–10 minutes)

### Correct technique

- Follow instruction for preparation of device
- Normal breathing through mouthpiece or face mask
- Breathe continuously until mist no longer produced by nebulizer

## ULTRASONIC NEBULIZERS

Ultrasonic nebulizers produce the cloud by dropping the solution into a plate that vibrates at high frequency. They are expensive and unsuitable for some drugs (antibiotics, DNAse), which may be destroyed by the device. On the whole these devices have no advantage over the much cheaper jet nebulizers.

## CHOICE OF DEVICE

The actual dose of medication reaching the lungs from most devices is only about 10% of that nominally delivered by the inhalation device, whether it be an MDI, DPI or nebulizer, and in many situations it is even less. Much of the drug is impacted on the device itself; some particles are too large to reach the lungs and impact on the buccal mucosa, with the potential for systemic absorption. This is particularly important for inhaled steroids and there are some data to suggest that the use of a spacer reduces this unwanted effect. Even though the lung dose is relatively low, drug delivery by inhalation is usually highly effective if the correct technique is used.

For most COPD patients it is probable that multidose DPIs are the most suitable devices for inhaling glucocorticoids or $\beta_2$-agonists. Anticholinergic bronchodilators are now available in dry powder formulation and muco regulatory agents are available only for wet jet nebulization. Some patients will simply be unable to master the use of MDIs or DPIs and will be able to use only a wet jet-type nebulizer or an MDI and spacer. It is rare that a COPD patient will do well with an MDI alone.

**Remember**
- The doctor must know how to use the inhalation device he/she prescribes
- The patient must be taught how to use the device by someone who knows how to use it
- The use of the device by the patient should be carefully checked at clinic visits

# Bronchodilators

Bronchodilators (or relievers) give relatively rapid relief of symptoms and are believed to work predominantly by relaxation of airway smooth muscle (although several other effects on the airways may contribute to their therapeutic effects). They are the mainstay of management of COPD. The choice and doses of bronchodilators available in the UK are given in the Appendix.

## ANTICHOLINERGICS

Anticholinergics are the bronchodilators of choice for COPD and in many studies have been shown to be more effective than $\beta_2$-agonists. The most commonly used drugs are ipratropium bromide (MDI, DPI or nebulizer t.d.s. or q.d.s.) or oxitropium bromide (MDI t.d.s.).

### Mode of action

Muscarinic receptor antagonists inhibit cholinergic reflex bronchoconstriction and reduce vagal cholinergic tone, which is the main reversible component in COPD (Fig. 10). In addition anticholinergics may reduce mucus hypersecretion. There is no effect on pulmonary vessels, and therefore no fall in $Pa,O_2$, as may sometimes be seen with $\beta_2$-agonists.

### Recommended use

Regular treatment is with MDI, DPI or nebulizer t.d.s. or q.d.s. Combination inhalers with an anticholinergic and a short-acting $\beta_2$-agonist are useful in some patients, giving a greater speed of onset of action and additive bronchodilator effects.

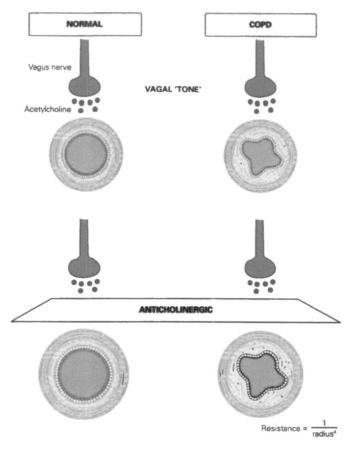

**Figure 10** *Mechanism of action of anticholinergics. Vagal tone has a greater effect in structurally-narrowed airways in COPD compared to normal airways, as airway resistance is proportional to 1/radius⁴. Anticholinergic drugs which block the vagal tone therefore have a bronchodilator effect.*

## Side-effects

- Paradoxical bronchoconstriction (usually due to additives in nebulizer solution)
- Glaucoma (especially with nebulized drug when used without mouthpiece)

- Bitter taste
- Systemic effects such as dry mouth, urinary retention, or constipation (very rare)

## SHORT-ACTING INHALED β₂-AGONISTS

## Mode of action

- β₂-receptors on airway smooth muscle: relaxation in large and small airways
- Functional antagonists: reverse bronchoconstriction irrespective of cause
- Have been shown experimentally to reduce plasma exudation and cholinergic reflexes
- Increase mucociliary clearance
- No effect on chronic inflammation

## Recommended use in COPD

There is immediate relief of symptoms. Ideally β₂-agonists should not be used regularly (there can be tolerance of the protective effects), although in patients with severe COPD regular nebulized β₂-agonists may be indicated.

## Side-effects

- Muscle tremor (direct effect on skeletal muscle β₂-receptors); more common in elderly patients
- Tachycardia (direct effect on atrial β₂-receptors, reflex effect from increased peripheral vasodilatation via β₂-receptors)
- Hypokalaemia (direct effect on skeletal muscle uptake of K⁺ via β₂-receptors); usually a small effect
- Restlessness
- Hypoxaemia (increased V/Q mismatch due to pulmonary vasodilatation)

## LONG-ACTING INHALED β₂-AGONISTS

Salmeterol and formoterol give bronchodilatation and protection against bronchoconstriction for more than 12 hours. There is increasing evidence that these drugs are useful as additional bronchodilators in patients with COPD and should be considered as supplementary to anticholinergics.

## ORAL β₂-AGONISTS

Although inhaled $\beta_2$-agonists are preferred, some elderly patients have problems with inhalers. Slow-release oral $\beta_2$-agonist preparations, such as bambuterol and slow-release salbutamol, are available. The advantage of these preparations is that they may treat peripheral airways more effectively, but the disadvantage is that side-effects are much more frequent than with inhaled preparations.

## THEOPHYLLINE

Theophylline is a useful additional bronchodilator in patients with COPD and oral administration has the advantage of treating small airways. It may have additional properties such as effects on mucociliary clearance and on respiratory muscles that are useful. The major limitation to the use of theophylline is side-effects.

## Mode of action

- Phosphodiesterase inhibition (increases cyclic AMP and cyclic GMP levels): important for bronchodilator action
- Adenosine receptor antagonism (accounts for some of the side-effects, but little evidence of relevance for bronchodilator effects)
- Increased adrenaline (epinephrine) secretion (but unlikely to account for effects in COPD)
- Prostaglandin inhibition
- Inhibition of calcium entry/release or phosphoinositide hydrolysis
- Unknown: difficult to explain all of the beneficial effects of theophylline on above mechanisms, as many only occur at concentrations higher than those used therapeutically

## Recommended use

This is recommended as an additional bronchodilator in patients not controlled on regular inhaled anticholinergics. It is useful in patients who have problems at night. A slow-release preparation should be given twice daily, with a higher evening dose to give steady state plasma concentrations of 10–20 mg/litre.

## Side-effects

- Nausea and vomiting
- Headache
- Restlessness
- Gastro-oesophageal reflux
- Diuresis
- Cardiac arrhythmias (usually plasma concentration >20 mg/litre)
- Epileptic seizures (usually plasma concentration >30 mg/litre)

## Clearance of theophylline

The therapeutic effect is related to plasma concentration, which is affected by several factors that alter clearance. If there is doubt, plasma concentration should be measured.

### Increased clearance (increase dose)

- Enzyme induction (rifampicin, phenobarbitone, ethanol)
- Smoking (tobacco, marijuana)
- Childhood
- High protein, low carbohydrate diet
- Barbecued meat

### Decreased clearance (decrease dose)

- Enzyme inhibition (cimetidine, erythromycin, ciprofloxacin, allopurinol, ketoconazole)
- Congestive heart failure
- Liver disease
- Pneumonia
- Viral infection and vaccination
- High carbohydrate diet

# Antibiotics

Since infection is so often the cause of progression or acute deterioration in patients with COPD, the combating of infection by the appropriate use of antibiotics is an important part of therapy. In fact, the organisms causing pulmonary infections are often the same as those found normally in the upper respiratory tract; it may be difficult to know whether a pathogen isolated from the sputum is responsible for the exacerbation. For most of the time the sputum in COPD is mucoid, but it becomes yellow or green with exacerbations of infection. When this occurs it is usual to begin empirical antibiotic therapy. The same applies to an exacerbation which manifests itself as increased breathlessness, increased cough or new changes in the chest radiograph.

The usual organisms responsible for exacerbations of COPD include:

- *Streptococcus pneumoniae*
- *Haemophilus influenzae*
- *Moraxella catarrhalis*
- Mycoplasma (less common)
- Viruses (increasingly recognized)

The choice of antibiotic depends upon:

- The likely organisms
- The likely sensitivity of the organisms in the community
- The tolerance of the patient for the drug
- The response to treatment

The treatment of choice in the community will often be either amoxycillin or trimethoprim/sulphamethaxozole (Septrin). However,

because many strains of *H. influenzae* are now β-lactamase pro-
ducers and hence resistant to ampicillin/amoxycillin, the treatment
for initial therapy commonly lies among:

- Amoxycillin/clavulanic acid (Augmentin)
- Erythromycin
- Cefaclor
- Doxycycline
- Clarithromycin
- Azithromycin

Table 5 gives an approximate breakdown of the sensitivities of the
common organisms found in COPD to these drugs.

There are advantages and disadvantages to each drug and the
choice may finally be based on finding out 'what works' for a given
patient. Cost is also a factor; there is no justification for using an
expensive drug when a cheaper one works just as well. In most
cases, the choice usually falls between amoxycillin,
amoxycillin/clavulanic acid or doxycycline for the typical ambulatory
patient.

|  | S. pneumoniae | H. influenzae | M. catarrhalis |
|---|---|---|---|
| **Amoxycillin** | S | S/R | R |
| **Amoxycillin/ clavulanic acid** | S | S | S |
| **Erythromycin** | S | P | S |
| **Cefaclor** | P | P | P |
| **Doxycycline** | P | P | S |
| **Trimethoprim/ sulphamethoxazole** | P | S | S |
| **Clarithromycin** | S | P | S |
| **Azithromycin** | S | P | S |

**Table 5** *Sensitivities of common organisms in COPD. S, fully sensitive; P, partially
sensitive; R, resistant.*

The antibiotic should be given in full therapeutic doses for a course
lasting about 10–14 days, except for clarithromycin and

azithromycin, which are given for shorter periods. Treatment is then stopped, provided the patient has responded. If there has been a poor response a change of antibiotic may be indicated, usually to one of the newer broad spectrum agents such as clarithromycin, if this has not already been tried. Continuous antibiotic administration is not recommended in COPD, as this has not been shown to alter the course of the disease.

# Other drug therapies

Although bronchodilator therapy is the mainstay of treatment in COPD, other treatments are commonly used.

## STEROIDS

COPD is defined by a lack of response to oral steroids in a short-term trial. In many patients of formal *trial of steroids* is important to exclude chronic asthma. The role of inhaled steroids in COPD patients is still not yet certain. Anecdotally, some patients seem to do well, and in some studies improvement in exercise tolerance has been demonstrated. However, no effect of long-term inhaled steroids on lung function or airway responsiveness has been found. Three large controlled trials have shown that inhaled steroids do not reduce the long-term decline in lung function. Inhaled steroids may reduce the severity of exacerbations and a three month trial of inhaled steroids may be given to patients with severe COPD who have frequent exacerbations. Inhaled steroids are also indicated when a trial of oral steroids is positive. Other patients should *not* be treated with inhaled steroids as there is a risk of systemic side effects with high doses in a susceptible population (elderly, immobile and often with a poor diet).

*Cromones* (sodium cromoglycate and nedocromil sodium) have no role in the management of COPD.

## MUCO REGULATORY AGENTS

Because mucus hypersecretion is a prominent feature of chronic bronchitis, various mucolytic therapies have been used to increase the ease of mucus expectoration, in the belief that this will improve lung function.

- *Stopping smoking* is the most effective way to reduce mucus hypersecretion.
- *Anticholinergics* may decrease mucus hypersecretion.
- *$\beta_2$-agonists* and *theophylline* may improve mucus clearance.

*Steam inhalation* (with or without aromatics) may provide symptomatic relief, but there is no evidence that it improves lung function or long-term symptom control.

Several drugs, such as *carbocisteine*, *bromhexol* and *ambroxol*, reduce mucus viscosity in vitro, but there is little evidence from controlled trials that they improve lung function in patients with COPD, and they cannot be recommended as routine therapy. However, some published studies have shown a reduction in the number of exacerbations.

Expectorants, such as *guanifeniesin* and *potassium iodide*, similarly have no proven beneficial effects.

*Recombinant human DNAse* (Pulmozyme) has beneficial effects in some patients with cystic fibrosis, but its role in COPD is not yet clear. Until there is clear evidence of benefit in COPD it should not be used in view of its high costs.

## ANTIOXIDANTS

Since oxidant damage may be critical in the pathophysiology of COPD, antioxidant therapy is logical. *N*-acetyl-cysteine was originally developed as a mucolytic, but has well documented antioxidant effects. Controlled trials have demonstrated that it reduces the frequency and severity of acute exacerbations of COPD and significantly reduces the rate of decline in lung function. It may therefore be useful in long-term management of COPD, but is not currently available on prescription in the UK.

## TREATMENT OF DYSPNOEA

Breathlessness is a problem in many patients, particularly 'pink puffers'. Several drugs, including opiates and benzodiazepines, reduce the sensation of dyspnoea but the reduction in ventilatory drive is potentially dangerous and these drugs are best avoided, particularly during exacerbations.

## RESPIRATORY STIMULANTS

There is no role for respiratory stimulants, such as doxapram or almitrine, in the long-term management of COPD.

## PREVENTION OF INFECTION

Immunisation against influenza is recommended for all COPD patients who have exacerbations. There is no evidence yet that vaccination against Pneumococcal infections is helpful in COPD. The recently introduced drug, zanimivir, is a neuraminidase inhibitor which prevents and reduces the duration of influenza. Although patients with COPD are likely to benefit, this has not yet been demonstrated in controlled trials.

# Oxygen therapy

Poor oxygenation is one of the fundamental problems of COPD and supplementary oxygen has long been part of therapy. Controlled oxygen is used acutely in the treatment of acute exacerbations. Long-term oxygen therapy (LTOT, domiciliary oxygen) is indicated in certain patients with COPD.

Two large multicentre trials have demonstrated that long-term oxygen administration (>15 hours daily) prolong survival (by about 30%) in patients with COPD.

## EFFECT OF SUPPLEMENTARY OXYGEN

- Improvement in exercise capacity (increased endurance)
- Reduction in dyspnoea
- Reduction in pulmonary hypertension, by reducing hypoxic pulmonary vasoconstriction
- Reduction in haematocrit, by reducing erythropoietin levels
- Improved quality of life and neuropsychiatric function

There are three methods of providing domicillary oxygen therapy:

- Long-term, low-dose oxygen (LTOT) for patients with chronic respiratory failure
- Portable oxygen therapy for exercise-related hypoxia and dyspnoea
- Short-burst oxygen therapy for temporary relief of symptoms

## SELECTION OF PATIENTS FOR LTOT

In the UK, guidelines have been drawn up for the provision of LTOT (Department of Health 1985). *LTOT should never be considered in patients who continue to smoke.* All patients should be assessed by a pulmonary specialist.

**Absolute indications:**
- Stable COPD over 3 weeks with hypoxaemia and oedema *and*
- FEV, <1.5 litre, FVC <2.0 litre *and*
- $Pa_1O_2$ <55 mmHg (<7.3 kPa), $Pa_1CO_2$ >45 mmHg (>6 kPa)

**Relative indications:**
- As above but without oedema or $Pa_1CO_2$ >45 mmHg

**Palliative (symptom relief):**
- To reduce severe breathlessness in terminally ill patients

*Portable oxygen* is indicated in patients who desaturate during exercise. Its efficacy needs to be assessed during a treadmill or 6 minute walk, patients wearing the portable oxygen cylinder. Portable oxygen may also be indicated in patients with severe exercise limitation irrespective of oxygen desaturation. *Portable oxygen may also be needed in such patients during commercial airline flights (provided by airline).*

## OXYGEN SUPPLY

There are several ways of providing supplementary oxygen:

- *Compressed gas cylinders* containing 100% $O_2$ are inconvenient, as regular delivery is needed and the cylinders are large and heavy, but this is still the most widely used method in the UK. Fitted with flow meters that are either medium (2 litres/min) or high (4 litres/min)
- *Liquid oxygen* is the most portable but most expensive form of supplementary $O_2$. Lightweight devices weighing 3 kg can deliver $O_2$ for 14 hours at 2 litres/min
- *Oxygen concentrators* are the most economic and convenient way of delivering LTOT at home

Oxygen may be delivered by several devices:

- *Face masks:* tight fitting masks are the most efficient devices, but are uncomfortable and inconvenient for long-term use
- *Nasal cannulae* are the most commonly used means of $O_2$ delivery and usually have no problems. A flow of 1.5–2.5 litres/min is usually adequate to achieve a $Pa_1O_2$ of >60 mmHg (>8 kPa)

- *Transtracheal catheter:* transtracheal oxygen therapy (TTOT) may be useful in some patients who cannot tolerate face masks or nasal cannulae, but catheters have to be removed and cleaned frequently
- *Pulsed delivery systems* use a thermistor or pressure valve to deliver $O_2$ only during the beginning of inspiration. These devices are expensive but reduce the amount of oxygen used by over a third

# Management of complications

Some patients have many attacks of acute infection without ever developing respiratory failure or cor pulmonale, and others seem to progress inexorably on to cor pulmonale – the 'blue bloater' type of COPD. Since respiratory failure is often precipitated by an acute exacerbation of COPD and since cor pulmonale similarly often develops against a background of chronic respiratory failure, these conditions and their management are inevitably interrelated.

## ACUTE EXACERBATIONS

### Clinical features

- Increase in cough and sputum
- Purulent sputum
- Increase in breathlessness
- Increase in hypoxia
- Possible new infiltrates on chest radiograph
- Increase in airways obstruction measured by spirometry
- Fever not common or at most low grade

### Causes

- Infection of the respiratory tract
- Pulmonary embolism
- Spontaneous pneumothorax
- Inappropriate oxygen administration
- Drugs (hypnotics, tranquilizers, etc.)

## Management

- *Absolute ban on smoking* (if patient still smokes)
- Start of course of *antibiotics*
- Increase (or start) inhaled $\beta_2$-agonist and anticholinergic *bronchodilator – given 3–4 times daily by MDI with spacer or jet nebulizer*
- *Chest physiotherapy* or self-administered physiotherapy to mobilize sputum
- *Oxygen* if patient is significantly hypoxic at rest ($Sa_2O_2$ <90%)
- *Course of oral steroids* as this reduces the length of exacerbations and shortens hospital stay
- *Follow up* to be sure patient has improved

## CHRONIC RESPIRATORY FAILURE

## Clinical features

- Often develops insidiously and may be undetected in COPD
- $CO_2$ retention with persistently elevated arterial $P_iCO_2$ ($Pa_iCO_2$)
- Metabolic compensation with elevated plasma bicarbonate and base excess (BE) and relatively normal pH
- Hypoxia which may be disproportionate to elevated $Pa_iCO_2$ because of concomitant ventilation/perfusion mismatching in the lungs
- May become worse during sleep
- May be associated with mental confusion if severe
- Often leads to cor pulmonale
- Patients may underventilate when given oxygen because breathing is largely controlled by hypoxia

## Management

- Basically same as management of COPD
- Increase efforts to improve ventilation
- Treat infection – try to isolate pathogen
- Try to mobilize sputum
- Treat cor pulmonale if present
- Follow $O_2$ saturation and check $Pa_iCO_2$ periodically

- Home nasal intermittent positive pressure ventilation (NIPPV) has recently been shown to be very effective
- Respiratory stimulants (almitrine) are not indicated, as ventilatory drive is already maximal

## ACUTE RESPIRATORY FAILURE

## Clinical features

- Often develops on basis of chronic respiratory failure due to infection or some other complication such as pulmonary embolism or pulmonary artery thrombosis
- Patient becomes more hypoxic with cyanosis
- Underventilation causes rising $Pa,CO_2$ and falling pH
- Patient becomes confused and drowsy
- Patient becomes tired and ventilation deteriorates further
- Consciousness may be lost and respiratory arrest ensues

## Management

- First priority – ensure adequate but not excessive oxygenation – arterial saturation about 85–90%
- Treat COPD with bronchodilators, physiotherapy and antibiotics
- Monitor condition closely, including $Pa,CO_2$

*Patient improving:* continue treatment

*Patient deteriorating,* with progressive rise in $Pa,CO_2$, fatigue and/or confusion:

- Start planned assisted ventilation (BIPAP) if possible; if not, intubate and ventilate
- Once ventilated effectively sedation may be given to allow patient to rest
- Reduce $Pa,CO_2$ slowly over 24–48 hours by ventilation to reasonable levels (usually to normal $Pa,CO_2$ level for patient plus about 5–10 mmHg)
- When blood gases satisfactory, patient conscious, try extubation or stopping BIPAP and follow clinical state and arterial blood gases

*Patient improving:* continue treatment

*Patient deteriorating:*

- Re-institute mechanical ventilation
- Consider possible need for prolonged home ventilation

## COR PULMONALE

This appears as a complication of COPD and is due to the effect of disease and chronic hypoxia on the pulmonary vasculature.

## Clinical features

- Oedema of ankles
- Elevated venous pressure in the neck veins
- Prominent pulmonary second heart sound on auscultation (difficult to hear)
- Crepitations at lung bases
- Cardiomegaly on chest radiograph
- ECG showing P-pulmonale in lead 2 and right ventricular hypertrophy
- Echocardiography showing enlargement of right ventricle, pulmonary hypertension and sometimes reduced right ventricular ejection fraction

## Management
This is based on three elements:

**Treat basic disease with optimum therapy:**
- Antibiotics
- Physiotherapy
- Bronchodilators (theophylline may have value in addition to other drugs)

**Ensure adequate oxygenation 24 hours per day:**
- Beware of rising $Pa,CO_2$ and possible need for ventilatory support

**Use diuretics to reduce fluid retention:**
- Beware of possible hypokalaemia and hypochloraemic metabolic alkalosis

ACE inhibitors (captopril, elalapril) may be useful. Digoxin is indicated only if there is coexistent atrial fibrillation. Vasodilators may be hazardous as they lower systemic as well as pulmonary blood pressure.

# Surgery

There is a long history of surgery for COPD. Previously used techniques included vagal nerve section and carotid body surgery (to reduce breathlessness), but there was no convincing evidence for benefit.

## LUNG TRANSPLANTATION

Originally heart–lung transplantation was used in patients with end-stage emphysema, but more recently single lung transplantation (SLT) has become the favoured technique in view of the scarcity of donor organs, since this enables two patients to receive transplants from one donor. Most patients with emphysema do well with a single lung transplant, as the large majority of ventilation and blood flow goes to the transplant and not the remaining native lung. However, if there is likely to be severe residual infection in the native lung, or if it contains extensive bullous disease, heart–lung transplantation or preferably bilateral sequential SLT is preferred.

### Patient selection

- Upper age limit of 60 years is usually used
- Patients with a life expectancy of <18 months, or onset of cor pulmonale
- Recurrent or persistent sepsis and bilateral extensive bullous disease are contraindications to SLT
- Previous thoracic surgery is a relative contraindication (haemorrhage)
- Good renal and hepatic function are important
- Right ventricular failure is not a contraindication
- Psychological factors and a supportive family are important

## Complications

- Lung infection (opportunistic infections due to immunosuppression)
- Acute injection (confirmed by transbronchial biopsy)
- Chronic rejection (obliterative bronchiolitis)

## Prognosis

- 10–15% early mortality due to sepsis or diffuse alveolar damage
- 1-year survival 70–75%, 3-year survival 60%
- Marked improvement in quality of life and lung function ($FEV_1 \sim 50\%$ predicted with SLT)
- 30% develop obliterative bronchiolitis within 5 years

## Bullectomy

There is still controversy over the indications for bullectomy and good results depend on careful patient selection. The ideal patient is young with large bullae and minimal airway obstruction. In patients with COPD the problem is that surgical removal of one bulla leads to growth of other bullae as the emphysematous lung expands. Favourable features are large bullae ($>1$ litre) with demonstration of surrounding lung compression and a lack of generalized emphysema demonstrated by computerized tomography and a normal $K,CO$.

### LUNG VOLUME REDUCTION SURGERY

Recently reduction of lung volume by excision has become popular for the treatment of widespread emphysema, particularly in North America. This involves resection of peripheral portions of both lungs using novel stapling techniques to prevent air leaks. The intention is to allow the remaining lung tissue to ventilate more effectively and in carefully selected patients there is increased elastic recoil and a substantial improvement in lung function. Given the problems associated with lung transplantation this palliative procedure provides a realistic alternative for many patients. Careful patient selection is critical.

The patients who do best are those with localized areas of emphysema.

# Future trends

There have been relatively few advances in the therapeutic options for the treatment of COPD, but better understanding of the molecular mechanisms involved in the pathogenesis of COPD will undoubtedly lead to improved therapies in the future.

## NEW TECHNOLOGIES

Artificial ventilation devices have improved enormously. Noninvasive ventilation using *nasal intermittent positive pressure ventilation* (NIPPV) has been an important advance in the management of acute exacerbations of COPD in hospital. NIPPV corrects the hypercapnia and respiratory acidosis, while resting the respiratory muscles. Excellent results in management of acute exacerbations have been reported, with significant reduction in mortality and time spent in hospital.

## EARLY DETECTION

One of the most important developments in the future will be the detection of COPD at an earlier stage before symptoms appear. This will depend on screening of cigarette smokers in the community and instituting preventive measure (smoking cessation plans and possible drug therapy). More rigorous attempts to prevent smoking, particularly in teenagers, are needed, with a complete ban on cigarette advertising and increased taxation on tobacco. In the future it may be possible to detect the genetic polymorphisms that predetermine whether a patient will develop COPD with cigarette smoking. The development of small lungs in neonates, owing to malnutrition and smoking in pregnancy, may increase the risk of COPD in cigarette smokers and emphasizes the importance of trying to prevent cigarette smoking in pregnant women.

## $\alpha_1$-antitrypsin replacement therapy

Replacement therapy with human recombinant $\alpha_1$-antitrypsin has now been developed but this treatment, which requires repeated intravenous infusions or aerosol, is extremely expensive and may be indicated only in patients with homozygous $\alpha_1$-antitrypsin (Pizz) deficiency. This therapy is not yet available in the UK. In the future, gene therapy with replacement of the $\alpha_1$-antitrypsin gene may become feasible.

## New anticholinergics

Tiotropium bromide is a new long-acting anticholinergic drug, which has a duration of 24 hours and some selectivity for the muscarinic receptors in airway smooth muscle. Clinical trials of the drug have been very promising in COPD patients as it produces long-lasting bronchodilatation. Other selective anticholinergics are also being developed.

## Enzyme/mediator inhibitors

Specific *neutrophil elastase inhibitors* have now been developed and may be useful in preventing progression of emphysema, as neutrophil elastase is likely to be very important in its pathogenesis (although it is not the only protease involved). The cytokines interleukin-8 (IL-8) and tumour necrosis factor-$\alpha$ (TNF$\alpha$) may play a key role in recruitment of neutrophils into the lungs, and specific IL-8 and TNF antagonists are currently being developed. Release of oxygen-derived free radicals, such as superoxide anions, may also play an important role in the pathophysiology of COPD, and antioxidants may be an important approach to treatment in the future. New and more potent antioxidants are currently in development.

## Anti-inflammatory treatment

This has an uncertain place in the long-term management of COPD. The neutrophilic inflammation that characterizes COPD appears to be steroid-resistant. It is possible that other anti-inflammatory drugs, such as phosphodiesterase (PDE) type 4 inhibitors, might be effective, as these drugs, unlike glucocorticoids, inhibit neutrophils. Preliminary studies have demonstrated that

PDE4 inhibitors may give symptomatic and lung function improvement in patients with COPD, although doses may be limited by side effects such as nausea.

# Further reading

American Thoracic Society. Standards for the diagnosis and care of patients with chronic obstructive pulmonary disease. *Am J Respir Crit Care Med* 1995; **152:** S77–S120.

Anthonisen NR, Connett JE, Kiley JP, et al. Effects of smoking intervention and the use of an inhaled anticholinergic bronchodilator on the rate of decline of $FEV_1$. *JAMA* 1994; **272:** 1497–1505.

Barnes PJ. New therapies for chronic obstructive pulmonary disease. *Thorax* 1998; **53:** 137–47.

Barnes PJ. Molecular genetics of chronic obstructive pulmonary disease. *Thorax* 1999; **54:** 245–52.

British Thoracic Society. BTS guidelines for the management of chronic obstructive pulmonary disease. *Thorax* 1997; **52(suppl 5):** S1–S28.

Calverley P, Pride N. *Chronic Obstructive Pulmonary Disease.* (Chapman & Hall: London) 1996.

Lacasse Y, Wong E, Guyatt GH, King D, Cook DJ, Goldstein RS. Meta-analysis of respiratory rehabilitation in chronic obstructive pulmonary disease [see comments]. *Lancet* 1996; **348:** 1115–19.

Pauwels RA, Lofdahl CG, Laitinen LA, et al. Long-term treatment with inhaled budesonide in persons with mild chronic obstructive pulmonary disease who continue smoking. European Respiratory Society Study on Chronic Obstructive Pulmonary Disease [see comments]. *N Engl J Med* 1999; **340:** 1948–53.

Siafakis NM, Vermeire P, Pride NB, et al. Optimal assessment and management of chronic obstructive pulmonary disease (COPD). *Eur Respir J* 1995; **8**: 1398–1420.

Tarpy SP, Celli B. Long-term oxygen therapy. *New Engl J Med* 1995; **333**: 710–14.

Vestbo J, Sorensen T, Lange P, Brix A, Torre P, Viskum K. Long-term effect of inhaled budesonide in mild and moderate chronic obstructive pulmonary disease: a randomised controlled trial. *Lancet* 1999; **353**: 1819–23.

# Appendix: Doses of COPD medications

## BRONCHODILATORS

### Ipratropium bromide
Anticholinergic bronchodilator
*MDI* (20/40 µg/puff) 1–2 puffs 3–4 times daily
*Dry powder* (40 µg/puff) 1–2 or 3–4 times daily
*Nebulizer solution* (0.25 mg/ml) 0.25–1.00 ml 3–4 times daily

### Oxitropium bromide
Anticholinergic bronchodilator
*MDI* (100 µg/puff) 2 puffs three times daily

### Salbutamol
Short-acting β₂-agonist
*MDI* (100 µg/puff) with or without spacer 1–2 puffs as needed up to four times
daily
*Dry powder inhaler* (Diskhaler) (200 or 400 µg) 1–2 as needed up to four times
daily
*Nebulizer solution* (5 mg/ml) 0.5–1 ml diluted to 2–3 ml up to four times daily
*Slow-release tablet* (Volmax 8 mg) twice daily

### Terbutaline
Short-acting β₂-agonist
*MDI* (250 µg/puff) with or without spacer 1–2 puffs as needed up to four times
daily
*Dry powder inhaler (Turbuhaler)* (500 µg/dose) 1 inhalation up to four times daily
*Nebulizer solution* (10 mg/ml) 0.5 ml diluted to 2–3 ml up to four times daily
*Slow-release tablet* (prodrug bambuterol) 20 mg once daily

### Salmeterol
Long-acting inhaled β₂-agonist
*MDI* (25 µg/puff) 1–2 puffs twice daily
*Dry powder inhaler (Diskhaler)* (50 µg/puff) 1–2 puffs twice daily

### Formoterol
Long-acting inhaled β₂-agonist
*Dry powder inhaler* (6 or 12 µg/puff) 1–2 puffs twice daily

### Other β₂-agonists

These are available but used less often:
fenoterol, pirbuterol, reproterol, orciprenaline, rimiterol, tulobuterol

### Combination inhalers

Anticholinergic and short-acting β₂-agonist
*MDI:* Duovent (ipratropium bromide 20 µg + fenoterol 100 µg/puff) 1–2 puffs
3–4 times daily
*MDI:* Combivent (ipratropium bromide 20 µg + salbutamol 100 µg/puff) 1–2
puffs 3–4 times daily
Nebulizer solution: Duovent (ipratropium bromide 500 µg + fenoterol
1.25 mg/4-ml vial) one vial four times daily

### Slow-release theophylline preparations

Many preparations as prophylaxis
Build up to about 8 mg/kg twice daily with checks on blood level (N.B. These
doses are designed to give blood levels in the range of 10–20 mg/l)
Usually given as twice daily dose with a larger dose in the evening

## MEDICATIONS FOR ACUTE EXACERBATIONS

**Salbutamol**
Nebulized: 5 mg diluted to 2–3 ml with normal saline
*Intravenous:* initially 5 µg/min, then adjust to avoid excessive heart rate response (average 3–20 µg/min)

**Terbutaline**
Nebulized: 10 mg diluted to 2–3 ml with normal saline
*Intravenous:* 2.5–5 µg/min

**Ipratropium bromide**
Nebulized: To be added to β₂-agonist inhalation every 2–4 hours 0.5 mg (2 ml of 250 µg/ml solution)

**Prednisolone**
Oral: 60 mg stat, then tail down over 7–10 days

**Hydrocortisone**
Intravenous: 200 mg every 6 hours

**Methylprednisolone**
Intravenous: 100 mg every 6 hours

## MUCO REGULATORY AGENTS

NB Not prescribable on NHS

**N-acetyl cysteine**
*Oral:*                    200 mg three times daily

**Carbocisteine**
*Oral:*                    0.75–1.5 mg three times daily

**Methylcysteine hydrochloride**
*Oral:*                    100–200 mg 3–4 times daily

## COMMONLY USED ANTIBIOTICS

**Amoxycillin**
*Oral:*                    250 mg three times daily

**Co-amoxiclav (amoxycillin + clavulanic acid)**
*Oral:*                    250 mg three times daily

**Cefaclor**
*Oral:*                    250 mg three times daily

**Erythromycin**
*Oral:*                    250–500 mg four times daily

**Azithromycin**
*Oral:*                    500 mg once daily (3 days)

**Clarithromycin**
*Oral:*                    250 mg twice daily

**Co-trimoxamole**
*Oral:*                    960 mg twice daily

**Doxycycline**
*Oral:*                    100–200 mg daily

# NORMAL FEV₁ AND FVC VALUES

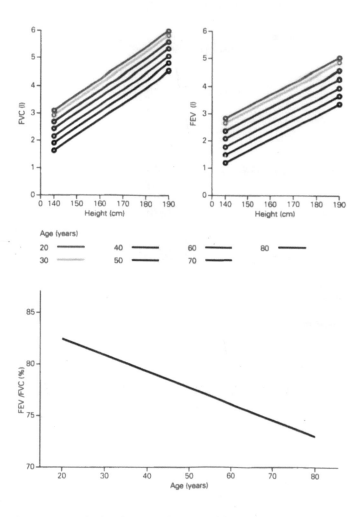

**Figure 11** *Normal values for FVC and FEV1 in adult men and their ratio to each other. From the Working Party on Standardisation of Lung Function Tests of the European Community for Steel and Coal. Eur Respir J 6: Suppl 16, 1993.*

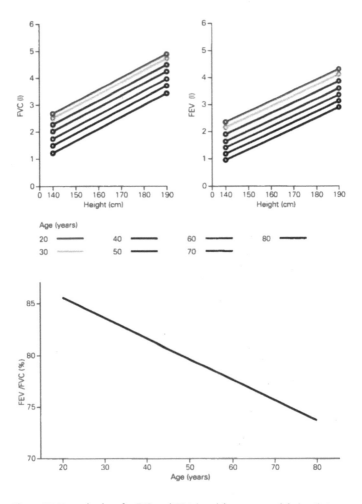

**Figure 12** *Normal values for FVC and FEV₁ in adult women and their ratio to each other. From the Working Party on Standardisation of Lung Function Tests of the European Community for Steel and Coal. Eur Respir J 6: Suppl 16, 1993.*

# Index